Nous Energy

Healing Power of the Pyramids

Glen-Martin Swartwout

A.B., B.D., O.D., N.D., F.I.C.A.N., F.C.S.O.

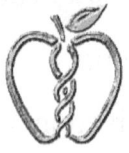

Published by Healing Oasis

Kingdom of Hawai'i

Other titles by Rev. Dr. Glen Swartwout

Refreshing Vision: Opening the Windows of the Soul

Cataract Solutions: Prevention & Reversal Via Accelerated Self-Healing

Healing Glaucoma

Macular Degeneration... ...Macular Regeneration

The Shire: Cultivating Your Future Self

Materia Medica: Vis Medicatrix Naturae

Electromagnetic Pollution Solutions

Biofields: The New Physics of Health

Table of Contents

Preface

In my work with the Remission Foundation, I come across many new and interesting health products. I utilize an electronic bio-communication process to observe how medicines affect all aspects of the body's physiology. For the first time in my 20-year career as a doctor, I have found a product that consistently treats the whole person, mind, body and spirit, accelerating the process of living, healing and learning to a new standard.

Dr. Glen

Summer 2001

Introduction

The purpose of this book is to share what clues are known about a first class medicine called Nouss-Ade. Though the medicine is no longer being produced, and remaining supplies are dwindling, the potency and significance of the observed healings and what can be learned in the process is as important now as it was when it was first discovered.

Welcome to the mysteries and the wonder of Nouss-Ade...

Dedication

This book is dedicated to Andrew Savva, who poured himself and some $13 million into the research and development of Nouss-Ade. He developed instrumentation to measure the nous energy fields and concluded that there is a tetrahedral (double pyramid) pattern of nous energy penetrating the earth's magnetic field. He identified a location in Australia where the energy matched that at Giza, and that is where he did extensive trials to find a way to stabilize that energy for healing purposes, ultimately finding that the mycelia of *Lentinula edodes* was the perfect carrier. From there, Andrew first brought his discovery in 2001, the year the Egyptian calendar ended, to Hawai'i, the site where a star tetrahedron or double pyramid resonance pattern inside the earth touches the surface, and the site of the largest and most active volcanoes on the planet. These are shield volcanoes, built like giant orgone accumulators... Andrew introduced his precious creation to this author, who had been brought to Hawai'i by the hereditary Kahuna of Pele's Heiau, a woman who, on the day she moved to Volcano Village in 1959, was greeted by a lava fountain that reached over 500 meters into the Heavens...

Nous Energy

There are no accidents.

Or as we say here on a regular basis... "Big Island... Small World."

Nous Energy

The discoverer of Nouss-Ade is an inventor, and also holds degrees in engineering, law and medicine. He has chosen to make this unique health catalyst available through select health practitioners who are prepared to enter into a new mode of health care. We are seeing life-changing results with Nouss-Ade on health, performance and longevity.

Nouss-Ade is a remarkable wellness product, having proven itself in Australia on over 100,000 patients. In the years of use by Remission Foundation clients around the world, we have seen that Nouss-Ade is a unique problem solving and healing-acceleration product you may want to use for life.

In the spontaneous remission of over 3,000 cases of cancer documented in the medical literature, a flu-like healing crisis is invariably part of the process as described in our interview, The Five Phases of Health produced several years ago with author, Kay Snow-Davis. This talk is very useful in understanding the various stages of the healing process experienced at an accelerated rate on Nouss-Ade.

To start experiencing the gentle yet profound energetic effects of Nouss-Ade personally, it is available with a retail price of $67.40 per bottle. Reports from Australia show that most professional people and those with chronic illness will want to maintain a level of two bottles a month long-term for enhanced energy, mental and physical performance as well as longevity. Nouss-Ade is one of those select few products that most people actually feel and want to keep handy.

On a personal note, I will share one final observation. Nouss-Ade is the first product I have found that has allowed one of my own family members to dramatically reduce the dosage needed of a top immunity product proven to triple NK cells. This has saved hundreds of dollars a month and at the same time providing new and dramatic healing benefits.

Foundations

The name Nouss derives from the Egyptian word nous for life energy, from the Greek nous, meaning mind. Other traditions have related concepts such as vital force, chi or prana. Virtually all life energy comes to earth from the cosmos, with life flourishing at the interface of earth's surface, which is exposed to this cosmic energy source from space.

The visible light spectrum supplies most of the energy of organic chemistry, but other energies are important, too. Far infrared waves penetrate deepest into the body's tissues, energizing minerals, stimulating circulation and melting fat. Near ultraviolet is essential in small amounts to produce Vitamin D from cholesterol in the skin, promoting immunity and reducing hip fractures by 50%.

Earth energies vary significantly over the earth's surface and are known to affect life and health. Geopathogenic zones, which are fluctuations in the earth's magnetic field, produce illness over time, while the Schumann field promotes health and balance. Now, some of the earth's most powerful geotherapeutic zones have also been mapped and this powerful healing energy has been stabilized in a capsule form.

Ancient scriptures refer to the "Elixir of Life," an energetic substance made up of the 5 essential energies vital for life on this planet, which in Eastern philosophy also make up both the heaven and earth chi. According to the investigations of Richard Hoagland, this knowledge may be a remnant of a golden age of science and technology that the Egyptians call "Zep-Tepi" or the First Time, which the Maya label as "the Fourth World," and the Greeks refer to as "Atlantis." In Tolkien's Middle Earth terminology, this was the First Age, or the Elder Days, when refined technologies like mithreal silver were know to Elven Science.

Oxygen Connection

Why is this energy so important to us today? One reason is that oxygen is a crucial link in the release of light energy from our food. Unfortunately, the atmosphere today contains only 20. 5% oxygen, and in cities and enclosed buildings that amount can sometimes drop to 10% or even 5%.

Evidence in air bubbles in both the polar ice caps and in amber (ancient pine sap) supports the notion that prior to the burning of fossil fuels during the past 300 years of the industrial revolution, earth's atmosphere contained 38% oxygen, a more optimal amount for maintaining our health and wellness.

Oxygen functions as a sponge for spent, low energy electrons and when it is deficient, high-energy electrons begin to escape the electron transport chain, damaging the cell structure. This is currently recognized as the common pathway of injury, aging and degenerative disease.

Body Electric

But even with adequate oxygenation, we need high-energy electrons to provide the vital force for optimum cellular life. The chemistry of life is largely an electronic process, as every chemical reaction is a transfer of electrons between atoms.

The vital force of each cell, 90% of which is generated in the mitochondria by oxidative phosphorylation through the electron transport chain, is expressed primarily at its cell membrane in an electrical force field much more concentrated than any technology currently known to mankind.

Nous Math

Sacred Geometry & Pyramid Connections

The limestone (calcite, CaCO3) pyramids of Egypt, along with the Great Wall in China and the Pentagon building are the only man-made structures visible to the naked eye from space. Calcite, the second most abundant mineral on the face of the earth after quartz (which some believe to have been used as a capstone on the pyramids), has a hexagonal symmetry (with right and left-handed hemihedron, rhombohedron, or scalenohedron shapes) with angles of 74 degrees 55 minutes between faces. Much of the limestone of the pyramids is composed of fossil shells and coral. We know that coral (largely composed of Calcium Carbonate or Calcite plus over 72 trace minerals) is associated with longevity when dissolved in drinking water. When the Guinness Book of World Records studied the oldest living man in 1979 in Tokunoshima, Japan, scientists identified the coral waters of the whole Okinawa Prefecture as the reason these islanders lived an average of 10 to 15 years longer than the rest of the Japanese population, when Japan itself already holds the record as the longest-lived nation in the world today. The effect of coral on water is alkalizing, antioxidant and provides trace minerals, which act as energy receivers and co-enzymes in the body. The mineral content of the pyramids (coral and shells concentrated into living organisms from sea water, which closely resembles the electrolytes of the blood), contains rare earth minerals that have been shown to extend the lifespan of laboratory animals by up to double. Coral and thus limestone and marble that it forms geologically are also found to be among the highest (along with volcanic sources) in m-state minerals, also known as ORMUS or orbitally rearranged minerals. M-state minerals are also associated with healing, longevity and seemingly miraculous effects such as levitation, bilocation, prophecy and other psi powers. M-state minerals are up to 4/9 non-local (out of space-time) and organize into a spatial matrix that can envelope biological systems. The electrons of these minerals cease to function as electrons and become bosons, or liquid light phonons that respond to thought, words and intent with a superconducting energy field that is immortal. This is a fourth state of matter known as a Bose-Einstein Condensate (BEC). The 5/9 of these minerals in space/time may be the part that translates and transcends the rest of the body (while still carrying its image) at the moment of death (as well as other out-of-body experiences or OBE's). Near death experiences often include a perspective of levitation as well as a sensation of intense blue or white light, which is also associated with angelic and m-state mineral healings. Precise measurements of body weight show a slight decrease at the moment of the soul's transition. M-state gold is the central goal of alchemy, which Nostradamus predicted would re-emerge by 1999, which in fact it did with David Hudson's patents. M-state rhodium and iridium form 5% of the brain's dry weight. The pharoahs, none of whose bodies have ever been found, were said to have made their transitions by taking a huge amount of m-state iridium and walking into the rising sun, disappearing in a flash of light, just as m-state iridium itself does. M-state minerals have very unusual properties, related to quantum mechanics, at a macroscopic level. They can be invited into presence. They respond to prayer and perserverence. They prefer to inhabit living organisms and protected niches in the environment. The move away from annoying electromagnetic interferences. The behave more like living, sentient beings like angels than other mineral states. M-state minerals generally appear as the minerals found in high levels in coral such as Calcium, Magnesium and Silicon, and some can take on the electrical appearance of Iron or Aluminum. Why were calcite pyramids built in the shape of huge magnetite crystal octahedrons? Why are they constructed with angles of 51 degrees 51 minutes and 51 seconds, which represents the Golden Mean ratio (phi or f=1.618:1 or 1:0.618), the only number series that is both an arithmetic and geometric progression, and is at the root of the structure of all matter? The Golden Mean is the ratio of the Fibonacci number series, which is:

0+1=1; 1+1=2; 1+2=3; 2+3=5; 3+5=8; 5+8=13; 8+13=21; 13+21=34

or 1, 2, 3, 5, 8, 13, 21, 34

with the ratios between numbers in the series of

2:1 = 2; 3:2 = 1. 5; 8:5 = 1. 6; 13:8=1. 625; 21:13=1. 615...1. 618...

The ratio between successive numbers more closely approximates the Golden Mean ratio as the number series continues.

Phi + 1 = Phi2

and also:

Phi = (1 + 5. 5) / 2

Why were these pyramids located where the huge stones had to be transported long distances for their construction? About 95% of the limestone used is made of jumbled seashells, with the nearest matching quarry located about 15 miles away, on the opposite side of the Nile river. Or, were they perhaps quarried from chambers fabled to exist beneath the plateau itself? The use of the pyramids as burial chambers appears to be more recent than their construction. Were these structures originally covered with gold (the most conductive metal) with a diamond (carbon) at the apex and were the chambers used for healing, leading later generations of Pharaohs to hope for eternal life by being buried there? Pyramid means "fire in the middle," like the fire in the middle of a person that is love. I believe that the pyramid acts a transmitter/receiver, an antenna and an amplifier of prayer, like the crystal in the original radios. We know that the pyramid shape itself, when located in the earth's electrical field, produces a negative ion field that promotes health, and even makes non-living objects like razor blades last longer (Czechoslovakian Republic Patent No. 91304 by radio and television engineer, Karel Drbal, 1959). In the 1930s, Antoine Bovis, a Frenchman, found a cat that had become naturally mummified in the King's Chamber of the Great Pyramid. It dried out even though the air is always at 80% humidity. He built a scale model of the pyramid in Paris and achieved similar effects with fruit and vegetables. According to Drbal, who began researching pyramid energy after reading Bovis' work, there is "A relation between the shape of the space inside a pyramid and the physical, chemical and biological processes going on inside that space." Did the builders of the pyramids have knowledge of the earth's natural sacred geometry guiding them to locate the site in Giza? They proved their knowledge of geometry by designing the pyramids based on the number:

Pi $=$
3.14159265358979323846264338327950288419716939937511...,

an infinite progression of numbers with no repetition, the ratio of a circle's circumference to its diameter, which has only been know in modern times for about 600 years. Clearly the builders of the pyramids also had some knowledge we lack even today, as current technology would be hard pressed to duplicate the construction of these massive man-made mountains, and other megalithic structures around the world. According to an experienced stonemason who researched many of the remarkable cut megaliths in Egypt, the type of fossilized limestone used requires two tons of pressure on a diamond bit to drill or cut. Also, it appears that the builders had knowledge of the earth's energy field as the pyramids were built in perfect alignment with the earth's magnetic field at the time of construction. It is unlikely that the pyramids were built originally as tombs, but other Egyptian tombs have been found with meals preserved well enough to identify every dish. Grains are preserved for thousands of years well enough that scientist have tried to sprout them. In contrast, our most modern grain storage silos can only hold grains a maximum of 4 years before they are destroyed by either fungus or insects. In the body, this is the equivalent of susceptibility to diseases produced by an imbalance in the ratio of electrons to protons. With too many protons, fungus grows. When electrons are in excess, parasites, bacteria and rapid aging occur. Did the ancient Egyptians who built these remarkable structures know how to balance subtle energies that could improve our prospects for health and longevity today?

The Shape of the Body

In Egypt today, Ibrahim Karim is researching biogeometry, finding that geometric shapes influence the growth of plants and can even allow crops to be grown when irrigated with seawater. When we think of our health, one of the most important features we talk about is what kind of shape we are in.

The pyramidal shape is a natural electro-acoustic resonator. The height of the pyramid is equal to the radius of a circle with a circumference equal to the perimeter of the square base of the pyramid, which is aligned to magnetic North.

The Great Pyramid of Giza is 481 feet high and 756 feet square at its base using some two and a half-million limestone blocks weighing 2 to 70 tons each cut to a tolerance of one-thousandth of an inch, but you can make a smaller pyramid to keep your razor sharp.... In Supernature – A Natural History of the Supernatural, author Lyall Watson says, "Cut four pieces of heavy cardboard into isosceles triangles with the proportion base to sides of 15.7 to 14.94. Tape these together so that the pyramid stands exactly 10.0 of the same units high. Orient it precisely so that the base lines face magnetic north-south and east-west. Make a stand 3.33 units high and place it directly under the apex of the pyramid to hold your objects. The sharp edges of the blade should face east and west. Keep the whole thing away from electrical devices."

After 10 years of study, metallurgists found that traces of water on the razor's edge made it dull while the pyramid removed the water by energizing it into a vapor. This means that the water affected by this energy carries higher energy electrons.

In 1968 American and Egyptian scientists recorded X-rays of the pyramid of Chephren, successor to Cheops in order to look for hidden vaults within the six million tons of stone. After running the X-rays constantly for over a year, an IBM computer analyzed the tapes, but they could find no pattern, even measuring from the same spot on different days. The project's leader, Amr Gohed, said, "This is scientifically impossible. Call it what you will – occultism, the curse of the pharaohs, sorcery, or magic, there is some force that defies the laws of science at work in the pyramid."

Later, in 1974, Stanford Research Institute attempted to map the inner structure of the pyramids using radio frequencies, only to find that the specific limestone used, combined with the 80% humidity in the structures led to total absorption of the radio-wave energy. Thus, the pyramids, to their surprise functioned as super-efficient radio-wave antennae and collectors (6 dB/m at 10 MHz to 25 dB/m at 150 MHz, proportional to the square root of the test frequency).

Dr. Paul Brunton, author of A Search in Secret Egypt, describes an out-of-body-experience while spending a night inside the King's Chamber. He was given a message to bring back to the world: "Know, my son, that in this ancient Temple lies the lost record of the early races of man and of the Covenant which they made with the Creator through the first of His great prophets. Know, too, that chosen men were brought here of old to be shown this Covenant that they might return to their fellows and keep the secret alive. Take back with thee the warning that when men foresake their Creator and look on their fellows with hate, as with the princes of Atlantis, in whose time this pyramid was built, they are destroyed by the weight of their own iniquity, even as the people of Atlantis were destroyed."

The Ark of the Covenant

The word ark comes from the Hebrew word aron, which means a chest or box. Its dimensions are described by the bible as 2.5 cubits by 1.5 cubits by 1.5 cubits (62.5 inches by 37.5 inches by 37.5 inches). Curiously, this is the exact volume of the stone chest or porphyry coffer in the King's Chamber in the Great Pyramid in Egypt. This coffer was the only object within the King's Chamber, as the Ark was the single sacred object within the Holy of Holies, in the Temple. Also the laver, or basin, that the priests used to wash their feet had the identical cubit dimensions. In addition, the cubit dimensions of the inner chamber of the Temple, the Holy of Holies, are precisely identical in size to the King's Chamber in the Pyramid and the same volume as the molten sea of water on the Temple Mount as prepared by King Solomon.

Since the Pyramid was built and sealed long before the days of Moses, when he built the Ark and the Holy of Holies, and had remained sealed for over twenty-five centuries until the ninth century after Christ, there is no natural explanation for the phenomenon of both structures having identical volume measurements. (Reference: Appointment with Destiny by Grant R. Jeffrey)

Nous Energy

A man born in Cyprus, Andrew Savva, of the Kiastor Clinic in Victoria, Australia claims to have cracked the code for the location of the pyramids. An engineer and inventor as well as a doctor and lawyer, this self-made man has traveled around the world on a spiritual quest, testing his own instruments and theories about cosmic energies and life.

Andrew's conclusion is that there is a tetrahedral (double pyramid) pattern of nous energy penetrating the earth's magnetic field. This energy concentrates most highly at five locations on the earth's surface, one of those being Giza. The others are in Australia, New Mexico, South Africa and South America. In each case, perhaps due to the intensity of this cosmic energy, the areas are now deserts.

Mycology & Medicine

One interesting feature, which Andrew has been able to identify is that the cosmic nous energy first penetrates all the way to the surface of the earth, and then radiates up to about 9 feet above the planet's surface as it mushrooms out in all directions, spreading its life-giving properties to the whole biosphere.

A tremendous amount of research around the world is documenting therapeutic properties in a number of mushrooms.

Lentinula edodes (shiitake): #1 therapeutic mushroom, anti-viral, anti-tumor.

Maitake: also contains beta glucans.

Cordyceps: athletes; fast recovery time.

Agaricus blazei: anti-cancer.

Reishi: immortality, detoxification, liver regeneration

Phellinus linteus: Anti-tumor (Korea).

Trametes versicolor: anti-cancer (in drug Kraston; Japan).

Hericium erinaceus: stimulates nerve growth.

Tremella mesenterica: anti-tumor; body tonic.

Pleurotus tuber-regium: Anti-tumor (Nigeria).

Pleurotus ostreatus: blood building, cholesterol lowering.

Inonotus obliquus: immune modulator (Russia).

Lepiota procera: (China).

Nous Energy

Flammulina velutipes: anti-tumor (Japan).

Many therapeutic mushrooms were grown at the site in Australia to discover one capable of storing the nous energy. At this site, in an area isolated about 200 miles from the nearest civilization, there is now a facility for growing, harvesting and processing the therapeutic mushroom, Lentinula edodes (shiitake), which millions of dollars and years of research has identified as having the capacity to store sufficient high energy electrons in its beta glucans to effectively transfer the nous energy for therapeutic purposes.

Similar effects have been documented with Kirlian photography, showing many times more light in the energy field of a fresh biodynamically grown carrot compared to a commercial product. The Bear study also showed that this difference could also translate into a 10,000% difference in beta-carotene levels. Even though both carrots looked orange, there was a 100-fold difference in nutritional value due to the conditions of growing and handling.

Once harvested at their maximum energy content, still in their early developmental stages prior to the opening of the gill slits and release of the reproductive spores, the juice of the mushroom buttons is dried and encapsulated, resulting in a 10 year stability
18

of the life-giving properties of this cosmically derived energy, a concentrated form of God's love for us, his beloved creatures.

Effects of Shiitake

Shiitake (Hua gu) has long been considered a medicine in the orient. Shiitake is known as the Monarch of Mushrooms, and at one time in Japan it was reserved for use by the emperor and his family. Over 2000 years ago, China's earliest materia medica describes more than 20 different species of mushroom including shiitake, out of the hundreds used in medicine today. During the Ming Dynasty era (A. D. 1368–1644), Chinese physician Wu Ri wrote about shiitake's abilities to increase energy, cure colds, and eliminate worms.

A native of the interior highlands of China, shiitake was the first mushroom to be cultivated some 1300 years ago in city of Qingyuan in Zhejiang province. Still today, Shiitake is the most frequently used therapeutic mushroom and Qingyuan is the world's largest shiitake producer with some 125,000 actively producing farms in the area.

In 1969, the government of Japan published a health survey showing that the two areas of Japan where shiitake was being grown, and also eaten more frequently, had a very low incidence of cancer.

The traditional dosage of whole, dried shiitake mushroom is 6–16 grams per day. Shiitake can occasionally trigger a temporary diarrhea and abdominal bloating if over 15 grams are taken in a day. For LEM, the dosage is 1–3 grams two to three times per day. Tinctures are also used at a dosage of 2–4 ml per day. With Nouss-Ade's potent energetic quality, only 200 to 600 mg are needed to achieve superior therapeutic results, or about 5% of the dosage of other forms. This indicates that the nous energy does about 95% of the healing work of Nouss-Ade.

Shiitake extracts approved for medical treatment in most countries include Lentinan, LEM, KS-2 and GVHR. Lentinan is found in the fruiting body, while Lentinula edodes mycelium (LEM) is rich in polysaccharides and lignans and is typically harvested before the stem and cap form. Laboratory studies indicate LEM has promise for those with HIV. KS-2 is a small protein-bound Alpha-Glucan that is readily absorbable. It is a metabolic byproduct of cultivating shiitake in a liquid medium.

Shiitake is typically grown on oak logs, taking up to 2 years to fully colonize a log before it begins forming fruiting bodies. Shiitake is said to be sweet, which relates to the Earth element

20

(digestion), neutral or balanced in temperature (neither hot nor cold), and slightly yang, or energizing. Regular use of shiitake is considered preventive for cancer and atherosclerosis, our culture's top killers.

Shiitake is now known to impart anti-fungal, anti-tumor and antiviral effects. Shiitake can even produce interferon. It has been recommended for Epstein-Barr virus (EBV) and for liver support. Shiitake is one of the few plant foods that supplies a high quality protein, with its 25-30% protein content providing all 8 essential amino acids in better proportions than soy, meat, dairy or egg. Shiitake is a particularly good source of glutamic acid. Shiitake also contains vitamins B complex, C, pro-vitamin D (more than any other plant) and E. Shiitake can lower high blood pressure, and also reduces cholesterol levels by up to 45%. It produces a compound that absorbs fat and helps promote needed weight loss.

Occasionally, minor cleansing reactions, such as skin rashes or diarrhea can occur with shiitake products. Hobbs also cautions those on blood thinning drugs to be cautious with shiitake as it may also tend to reduce blood clotting.

Chemistry of the Beta Glucans

Beta-Glucans are long chain polysaccharides with thousands or even millions of glucose molecules linked by covalent bonds at the beta (#2) sugar unit in each chain. Glucose is a 6-carbon (hexose) sugar ring, so the number of the carbon atom on each side of the linkage can also be specified, such as a 1-3 Beta-Glucan, which indicates that the #1 carbon of one glucose is bonded to the #3 carbon of the next. Side branches are noted in parentheses, such as (1-6) in 1-3 (1-6) Beta-Glucan found in shiitake, and patented as the world's leading primary anti-cancer drug Lentinan. Both Alpha and Beta-Glucans are found in shiitake and other therapeutic mushrooms.

Beta-Glucans attach to receptor sites on T cells, B cells and Natural Killer cells (NK cells), increasing both the number and activity of these cells. Within 3 days of starting Beta-Glucan supplementation, the active immune cell population can increase by up to 3000% to 5000%. This process is known as immunomodulation. Since infections cause more deaths in cancer patients than does cancer, Beta-Glucans are used world-wide as an adjunct to conventional treatments to help restore immune function lost to radiation and chemotherapy while supporting the immune system's direct anti-tumor effects.

In Japan, the complex sugar Lentinan was approved in 1975 and has become one of the top-selling anti-cancer drugs in Japan and the #1 worldwide. Instead of potentially cancer causing side effects, Lentinan is an immune modulator that can prevent the damage to chromosomes caused by many of the toxic synthetic chemotherapies. Evidence is mounting to show that Lentinan helps other chemotherapies to shrink tumors faster while reducing their side effects.

Lentinan is beneficial Hepatitis, and has been specifically documented on Hepatitis B.

Lentinan is also being studied as an adjunct treatment for HIV infection. When 88 HIV-positive people were given 2 mg Lentinan weekly in addition to the drug didanosine (400 mg per day), CD4 counts increased for a significantly longer period than without Lentinan. (Gordon M, Guralnik M, Kaneko Y, et al. A phase II controlled study of a combination of the immune modulator, lentinan, with didanosine (ddI) in HIV patients with CD4 cells of 200-500/mm3. J Med 1995;26:193-207.)

Clinical studies at Zhejiang University in Hangzhou, China, found chemotherapy only 10% effective for lung cancer, but achieved over 80% cure-rate with the addition of Beta-Glucans. Since

1994, this combination has been accepted as standard treatment in advanced lung cancer in China.

Another extract, eritadenine, is being studied for its potential to prevent heart disease risk by reducing blood lipids and cholesterol levels. According to Christopher Hobbs, L. Ac. , A. H. G. , writing in Medicinal Mushrooms (Botanica Press), shiitake may also improve liver function and help produce antibodies to hepatitis B.

A Japanese shiitake product, ImmPower, is now the top selling nutritional supplement in Japan. In America, ImmPower sells through doctors for $49.95 for 30 capsules. Another shiitake-based product developed by Dr. Mamdooh Ghoneum of Egypt (patent owned by Daiwa Pharmaceutical Co. of Tokyo), MGN3, a patented combination of rice bran and shiitake extracts, has been proven to triple Natural Killer (NK) cells and is used widely by those with such conditions as cancer, AIDS and hepatitis. The New England Journal of Medicine reported that giving Shiitake to patients with probable pre-AIDS improved their general condition and immune status.

Cancer patients taking MGN3 went into complete remission in a 7-month test, by taking 12 capsules a day. After two weeks, the immune system was destroying cancer cells 240% faster than

24

before, and this rate kept rising for six months. A test of 24 patients with a variety of different cancers found that their NK cells destroyed cancer cells 40% faster in just 16 hours, 800% in a week and 2,700% in 2 months. Clinical trials are also showing great results with HIV, AIDS, hepatitis, chronic fatigue syndrome (CFS), cervical dysplasia and other diseases. MGN3 is available in a double-strength caplet through doctors for $112.00 for 50. The regular strength is available in vegicaps as well as the original gelatin capsules for the same price of $62.95 for 50 capsules.

Shiitake Synergy

Taking about a gram of vitamin C, digestive enzymes and/or ginger (*Zingiber officinalis*) along with Beta-Glucans may enhance their digestion into smaller units that are more bioavailable.

Effectiveness

Over 100,000 people, mostly in Australia have already experienced the remarkable benefits of Nouss-Ade over the past 4 years. While no medical claims are being made for this remarkable food-energy supplement, the results clearly speak for themselves.

Nous Energy

Since adding Nouss-Ade to our clinic's range of over 5,000 natural products, individualized biofeedback analyses have found that over 36% of all our clients showed a marked therapeutic response to Nouss-Ade, making it the most frequently recommended product now in our repertoire.

The most remarkable feature of our clients' response characteristics to Nouss-Ade is its versatility as an adaptogenic supplement. It works as a problem solver to correct specific deficiencies and blockages in the most challenging conditions. It frequently balances up to 58% of the unbalanced meridians. The meridians most frequently balanced by Nouss-Ade are the Kidney, Neural (a.k.a. Nerval Degeneration Vessel), Gall-Bladder (which often reflects infectious and parasitic processes), Immune (a. k. a. Allergy Vessel in European Biological Medicine) and Large-Intestine.

To date, meridians balanced by Nouss-Ade, from the most frequently balanced to the least, are shown in the Meridian/Phase-Analysis chart below:

Meridian Balancing Effects of Nouss-Ade

Five Phase Analysis

System: Meridian: Cases: Phases:

1: Kidney: 38%: 22111112

4: Nerve: 38%: 11111114

3: Gall Bladder: 33%: 1114141

2: Immune: 29%: 111221

3: Large Intestine: 29%: 221122

2: Circulation: 24%: 21121

2: Heart: 24%: 42112

3: Stomach: 24%: 11211

4: Logic: 19%: 1121

3: Pancreas: 19%: 1221

4: Endocrine: 19%: 1111

2: Lymph: 19%: 2224

3: Lung: 19%: 2112

2: Fat Metabolism: 19%: 2214

1: Bladder: 19%: 4411

Nous Energy

3: Small Intestine: 14%: 212

3: Liver: 10%: 12

2: Joint: 10%: 11

2: Connective Tissue: 10%: 11

5: Skin: 10%: 12

4: Emotion: 5%: 1

2: Spleen: 5%: 2

Analysis of these electrodermal responses to Nouss-Ade by patients at the Hawai'i Center for Natural Medicine shows that while Nouss-Ade can balance functions and meridians in any phase, the most frequently balanced are Phase 1 and 2, the deepest, most serious health problems related to energy depletion, aging and degeneration. It is no wonder that people describe a feeling of immortality when supported with Nouss-Ade.

Five Element Analysis

Element: Yin, Yang, and Ratio

Water: 8: 4: 2

Wood: 2: 7: .3

Fire: 9: 8: 1.1

Earth: 5: 5: 1

Metal: 4: 6: .7

Five Embryological Tissue Layer Systems Analysis

System: #, Points, and %

System 1 (Flow): 12: 4: 14%

System 2 (Support): 29: 15: 9%

System 3 (Process): 31: 13: 11%

System 4 (Communicate): 17: 6: 13%

System 5 (Integrity): 2: 2: 5%

Totals: 91: 40: 11%

Analysis of these effects in the different tissue layers shows the greatest effect in the deepest layer, System 1, which includes the Kidneys, traditionally observed as the site where the jing or most precious ancestral essence is stored. Following close behind is the communication system, System 4, associated with the neuroendocrine functions and consciousness. In Oriental Medicine, the nervous system is also governed by the Water Element.

Study of 196 Nutraceuticals

Nutraceutical: NK Cell Increase

Noni (Morinda citrifolia): 15%

Aloe vera concentrate (acemannan): 15%

Endocrine System Formula: 16%

Phytonutrient Formula with Garlic: 21%

Bovine Colostrum: 23%

Cordyceps Formula: 28%

Shiitake mushroom: 42%

Echinacea: 43%

Plant Polysaccharide formula: 48%

IP6: 49%

4Life Transfer Factor: 103%

4Life Transfer Factor Plus (with shiitake): 248%

Other Shiitake-based products not included in this study:

MGN3 (with shiitake): 300%

ImmPower (with shiitake): no study yet; #1 supplement in Japan

Nouss-Ade (with shiitake): no study yet; very popular in Australia

As an example, K. Aubrey Niles, a wholistic therapist with whom I have worked for many years has been successfully using a therapeutic dose of double-strength MGN3 to overcome cancer. MGN3 in the regular strength has been documented to triple natural killer cell levels. With a retail cost of $448 per month, however, she has tried many promising alternative products with no success as a substitute.

Each time she reduced the dosage of MGN3, severe symptoms such as heart and liver pain, and swelling in multiple affected areas would ensue immediately. When she first took Nouss-Ade, there was clearly a dramatic shift in her healing process, and for the first time she is able to achieve a reduced maintenance dosage of MGN3, easily covering the cost of the Nouss-Ade. And even more importantly, her healing process is further accelerating.

Initially, for most people, a noticeable increase in energy and endurance is usually experienced, along with the restoration of natural youthful feelings including increases in libido, tightening of the skin, and a decrease in aches and pains. Most people also notice an increase in certainty in life and a greater connection with self and others.

I experience Nouss-Ade as an accelerator of life's purpose and meaning, as well as metabolism and healing. It is as though it

31

compresses the spiral of time, so that we are catapulted through life's processes by quantum leaps. When I go to make a choice, whether large or small, whether nutritional, social or economic, it is as though I am experiencing simultaneously the choice I contemplate and its end result, allowing me to more easily make only choices in alignment with God's will and my highest good.

In my own personal experience, this is obvious to me when I am able to make food choices, both in quality and quantity that in the past would have violated my own intellectual knowledge and understanding. Somehow, Nouss-Ade provides a specific and unique type of energy that fortifies the will, making its proper application virtually effortless. I believe this is a divine grace preparing us for a future in which we all live in harmony and union with God's plan for us.

My personal observations during the initial time taking Nouss-Ade are:

From first dose, bowel function improved to 3 bowel movements a day.

From day 2, morning swelling and irritation around hiatal hernia areas reduced by 90%. If I miss a few doses, it comes back.

From about day 4, I noticed a smile coming across my face in the morning as soon as I realized I was awake. This new joy in life also showed up in spontaneous singing around the house.

From the first week, I notice a profound shift in my ability to foresee the outcome of choices, such as how I will feel an hour after eating a sweet 'health-food' treat.

After about 2 weeks taking 2 capsules twice a day, when I missed taking Nouss-Ade for over 24 hours, I could clearly see an amazing contrast in energy level. I woke feeling heavy intertia, even more than I typically did before taking Nouss-Ade, as though it had been moving a lot of heavy metals out of my body with the enhanced elimination. This would fit what I know about my body. I took a Kirlian photo before and after taking the next dose and it showed a blocked energy pattern that began to unblock again within a half hour. I felt great again within a day. I decided to try taking just 2 capsules a day to slow down the detoxification process a bit.

From the first month, I definitely notice increased mental energy and focus. I am getting a lot more accomplished that I intend to do, and less time spent on procrastination/avoidance behaviors with insignificant details. I feel as though the energy in this product is allowing me to jump to the next performance level in my life. Since starting Nouss-Ade, I am now working on several major business projects simultaneously each of which should be able to fund my life's goals within a couple years or less. I am spontaneously becoming more of a team player, overcoming my life-long tendency toward personal control and the limitations of perfectionism.

After 2 months, I found myself achieving much more and wanting to take 3 to 4 capsules a day to support my energy needs. I feel that a good bulk of the detoxification is accomplished, although I am aware that these processes often do go in cycles, so I continue to monitor my desired dosage level. Clearly, though, my relationship with the Nouss-Ade has shifted from 'black smoke coming out the tail-pipe' to an experience of sustained high-test performance enhancement unparalleled with any other product I have tried, even those I have formulated myself, such as the popular energetic solutions Stamina Plus and Energessence, which are popular among professional athletes.

For anyone with an existing health concern, the therapeutic dose of Nouss-Ade is two capsules twice a day for the first four months. Maintenance of healthy aging and spiritual growth support is achieved with one capsule twice a day.

Another approach I often recommend is beginning with one capsule the first day and increasing by one capsule a day up to 4 to 6 total. This way you can find the level of acceleration that best suits you to begin with. It is like taking a vehicle that has been driving around town your whole life and taking it out on the freeway for the first time. You may experience some knocks and black smoke as you clear out the pipes and gradually clean out the build up that has accumulated over the years.

Nouss-Ade is unique in working on the spiritual/energetic side of causality, allowing the body's innate intelligence to divinely guide the healing and growth process.

Results

According to Michael J. Costar, H.D., Hb.T., of Essence of Life, "Nouss-Ade in my opinion has got to be the greatest scientific breakthrough in modern history. I have found that simply everyone that goes on this product finds they don't want to be without it. Why would this be the case? It is believed that in ancient times we received 'prana' universal life sustaining energy directly through our 'crown chakra,' which enabled our body cells to be nourished and maintained by these high levels of 'essential essence'. Today we only take in a limited amount of 'prana' via

35

the air we breathe and the food we eat. Due to our often-fast lifestyle & the stressed environment, we must work hard to maintain the ability to stay close to any level of wellbeing. Nouss-Ade thanks to a modern day miracle discovery, delivers to our bodies the precise level of 'prana' we need to maintain cellular energy levels sufficient enough to allow for optimum well being. The overall effect is an energized body, mind and spirit which given time, induces healing without exception, the very way nature intended. This indeed explains why people just want to have more. Nouss-Ade is truly an accomplishment almost beyond belief, but the proof of the pudding is in the eating…"

Len Bauers' Massage and Rejuvenation Centre reports, "Our feedback on the new Nouss-Ade capsule has been very positive indeed, so I have put together a quick report on some of the responses that we have received from different people, treating different problems.

Tiredness: Most are losing that dragging tiredness and waking up feeling brighter and refreshed.

Weight: Fantastic!!! Try as they might to eat the right diet, they finish up eating the wrong foods and yet weight keeps disappearing.

Pains: At times seem to decrease, at times seem to increase then stop.

Flatulence: For those who have it, it seems to have mellowed…

Bowels: For most there has been a major improvement.

Kidney Stones: Have been passed (these were not realized being there until passed).

Hemorrhoids: Profuse bleeding stopped immediately, coloured a couple of times and are no longer hanging around. GREAT!!!

Fluid Retention: Ankles are no longer swollen.

It is an honour to be promoting Nouss-Ade after trying so many different "band-aids". At this stage I give Nouss-Ade the 5 star.*****"

Many people report reduction of:

Arthritis
Asthma
Back pain
Chronic fatigue
Diabetes
Eczema

Nous Energy

Food consumption (by up to 2/3, which can cover the cost)

Gout

Heart problems

Herpes

Hunger

Impotence

Joint pain

Low energy

Menopausal symptoms

Menstrual pain

Migraine

Osteoporosis

Prostate cancer

Prostatitis

Psoriasis

Skin cancer

Stress

Barry Grundler compiled some of the results his clients achieved:

High Blood Pressure

Six (6) people with high blood pressure (160/100 or more) are now having normal reading of 120/80 since taking Nouss-Ade.

38

Kidney Problems

Three (3) people with kidney problems had been advised that they would require to be dependent on the dialysis machine in the near future and since taking Nouss-Ade, their tests at the hospital had shown improvements.

Arthritis

Three (3) people suffering from arthritis had advised on improvements since taking Nouss-Ade.

Eating Disorders

One person had suffered heartburn and shortness of breath as a result of craving to eat and since taking Nouss-Ade her craving had ceased and is now eating normally and also lost weight.

Diabetes

Two (2) people who are diabetic had experienced lack of energy and sleepiness but since taking Nouss-Ade they had found new source of energy and both enjoying almost normal life."

Learning Abilities

At age 15, Adam Stenning, born January 1st, 1985 writes, "I've been taking Nouss-Ade capsules for two years; they help me to concentrate in class; I wake up with more energy; I don't catch colds or the flu & I don't get pimples or acne."

Weight Loss & Weight Gain

Long Le decided to lose some weight for her wedding two years ago. Because she was skeptical, she only purchased one bottle of Nouss-Ade to start. She says, "Not only did I start to feel there was little need for food, I also felt an increase in energy level. I had eaten less food but still had the energy to exercise more often. I ended up losing lots of excessive weight in the 3 months prior to the wedding."

"Prior to taking the capsules, I had suffered from a flu in the previous 2 winters. The flu was so bad that I was twice bedridden, away from work. Since taking the capsules, I am a lot better and I feel protected every year."

"2 months ago, I decided not to order more capsules after they had run out. Strangely, I started to feel a sudden decrease in energy level, having worked 60 hour-weeks on a regular basis I become exhausted at the end of each day. As a result, I now continue to take 2 capsules a day and this has made a big difference to my life."

Michelle Trainer says, "I started 5 weeks ago and I have lost 5 1/2 kilo's in weight. I feel great I use to suffer with migraines but I have not had one in 5 weeks."

"I also put my daughter on Nouss-Ade. She has a life threatening muscle disorder. It is called Infantile Spino-Muscular Atrophy. She suffers with severe chest infections and spends most of her time in hospital. She took Nouss-Ade for 2 days and her chest is clear. Her physician can't believe it. Melissa is eating more and gaining weight. Since we have been taking Nouss-Ade I have started others on it. One lady has M. S. One young boy has Muscular Dystrophy and one young man has prostate cancer and diabetes and they are all feeling much better. I think everyone should take Nouss-Ade."

Healing

Lorri Buttner, one of the earliest users, has been taking Nouss-Ade for nearly four years. She reports "Last year I had two hip replacements as a result of a bad skiing accident many years ago. The replacements were 8 weeks apart and 9 weeks after that I embarked on a two-month walking holiday around Europe and Northern England. Surgeons, doctors and hospital staff were all amazed at my quick recovery and return of energy. Standing alongside people who had the same operation on the same day, it was clear to me also that my recovery was much faster."

Holy Grail of Health

Sherri McIver reports, "I was sold my first bottle of Nouss-Ade by a girlfriend in Queensland who spoke of it as the Holy Grail of Health. I really couldn't believe that something that came in such a daggy little bottle could achieve everything she claimed but was prepared to give it a go."

"I have since become a devotee, and although I still have no idea of what it is I'm taking, swear by it. I am a Yoga student and so remain a little skeptical that you can ingest Prana or 'life force' (we are taught that it comes in with the breath) but if that is what the people behind Nouss-Ade have achieved, then the whole world should be taking it."

"The health benefits I have noticed are an increase in energy and a marked improvement in digestion. The increase in energy is quite remarkable. I was someone who really 'faded' in the late afternoon but now find I can power on quite easily. I suppose the two are connected but an increase in waste elimination has also been very marked. Anyone who suffers from constipation (and the truth is, if you don't 'go' three times a day you're constipated) should take this product. I don't have any major health problems but find taking Nouss-Ade has increased my overall sense of wellbeing. It has given me the energy to undertake a major fitness overhaul and get on with all those things that are important to me."

Energy

Fiona Quayle, initially a skeptic, says, "All the benefits were explained to me and they gradually began to happen. Initially it was the energized way I felt. I was sleeping better and waking in a more refreshed frame of mind. I am epileptic [and] suffered from general tiredness and lethargy. The Nouss-Ade tablets did not cure me but gave me a more fulfilled and well-rounded life to live. My appetite was also reduced, which it needed to be."

Nous Energy

Sharon Forsyth of the Akasha Healing Center in Hawai'i reports "I have had kidney/adrenal exhaustion for several years now. I am still able to work, but I feel tired most of the time. I started on Nouss-ade in April. Within the first 3 days my energy level increased and a sense of effortlessness came over me. It was a different kind of energy than you may feel with stimulants, it was an expansive energy that also gave the body a boost."

Maureen Wharton writes, "When I commenced taking the product, my intention was to increase my energy levels, so that I could use my walking machine for longer than 2 minutes, as I had really packed on excess kilos over the last two years.

I have also suffered from a debilitating knee problem for the last 12 years.

To my surprise, after only 3 days, I was looking for an excuse to get off my machine after 15 minutes, but found that I still had not 'packed it in', which previously would have been another excuse to NOT walk. I then realized that the Nouss-Ade capsules had created this miraculous change for me. I have no more pain in my knee, and I can now walk as far as I want to without becoming puffed.

Another effect is that I have also lost 8 kgs."

CFIDS

"Thank you for giving me back my life!" writes Linda Condon, who was diagnosed with Chronic Fatigue Syndrome in 1995. After trying both medical and natural treatments from many doctors with little success, her sister shared a pamphlet on Nouss-Ade, which had helped a well-known sports figure in Australia. Though skeptical, she was willing to try one more time to find an alternative to being so weak that she had to be carried to the toilet. Neither Linda, nor her parents who had moved in to take care of her could believe it when after taking the first capsule of Nouss-Ade, she got out of bed and walked around.

Fibromyalgia

Jackie Levanic reports, "I now have a lot more energy in my daily routine. I feel a sense of peace not having to get up each day feeling 100 years old which is how I felt prior to taking Nouss-Ade. I was diagnosed with Fibro-Myalgia and Chronic Fatigue Syndrome quite some years ago and have not felt such relief from the symptoms of these diseases as received from taking Nouss-Ade. I have tried alternative medicines and conventional medicines but they have not come close to the relief I get when I take Nouss-Ade."

Subtle Healing

One family had taken Nouss-Ade for 10 weeks without noticing any benefits at all, but when asked about the child's constant illnesses, they realized the child was no longer prone to illnesses that had been a constant feature before. Their supplier reports, "When talking to the parents about others being helped, even addictions and cravings, the mother spoke up and said 'That's right I don't crave for chocolate anymore'.... People are not noticing their change to well being the body just starts asking for a better lifestyle and we take for granted."

Experience of a Physician

A medical doctor in Australia, Dr. Gill, was taking one capsule twice a day on and off over a period of a year. He reports, "When stopping the capsules I did not experience any withdrawal symptoms but my energy level and level of well-being seemed to slowly wane. Finally, about a month ago I decided to clarify the situation by increasing the dose to two capsules twice daily.... After increasing the dose I started to experience very significant changes within a day or so. I now realize that four capsules per day is the dosage that you recommend for people with some pre-existing ailment. In my case I found that there was a dramatic

46

increase in my energy levels. To my surprise I found myself unruffled in various situations, which would have normally been quite stressful. I seemed to have more stamina and sometimes finished my day's work still feeling fresh! Physically I felt a sense of well-being. My ear, nose and throat symptoms significantly diminished and I hope that they will eventually cease. My sleep pattern improved and became very refreshing and restful. I noticed that mentally there was much greater clarity and ease in my thinking. I write a lot of reports in my work and this is often a complex task. I found that I was able to formulate my thoughts and express them in the reports more clearly and with much less effort. All in all I have been very surprised and pleased at my improved feelings of energy and well-being since taking four capsules per day of Nouss-Ade."

Parkinson Symptoms

At age 62, Jeanne Dobson, who used to suffer from Parkinson's-like tremors, reports that "Nouss-Ade has been the most wonderful thing that has ever happened to me.... I'm not depressed any more, headaches are gone, my hair stopped falling out, my hormone levels are so much better, no more aches and pains, but the biggest thing is my head: no more shaking. I can put my head down on the pillow and sleep, no neck pain any more, I don't have to support my neck. It's a miracle.... I have just moved into a new home and have been able to design my garden, dig it, put in a vegetable patch, plant trees: I feel as strong as if I were in my thirties. Also my skin has improved dramatically: the lines are fading and it is lovely and soft.

Diabetes

Faith Kawaiti, age 63, has experienced failing health, including insulin-dependent diabetes, since a heart attack some 7 years ago. She has been unable to perform normal activities of daily living. She could not stand or walk without assistance and she could not even lie down without feeling dizzy and sick. She had also lost all feeling in her feet. A home-care nurse was required to administer about 15 prescription drugs twice every day and she was in and out of the hospital every two to three months. After a friend recommended Nouss-Ade, she started taking two twice a day for two weeks and then one twice a day for the following year. She reports, "During the time that I was on the Nouss-Ade capsules I noticed that my energy level increased dramatically. I found that I could breathe much easier, I could do the things that I needed to do around the house, I could lie down without getting dizzy so

I began to sleep well. Most importantly I did not need to go back to the hospital at all. This was an amazing change…."

Faith continues, "I discussed my improvement in my health with Dr. Owzinsky and told her that it was the Nouss-Ade that had caused my improvement. She told me to stop taking Nouss-Ade capsules as she said that she didn't know what was in them. I said to Dr. Owzinsky that she should contact Nouss-Ade but she said that she did not want to do that. She also told me that unless I stopped taking Nouss-Ade capsules she would stop to treat me."

"I also told the nurses that came to visit me about how much better I felt by being on Nouss-Ade capsules. One day a man, who I think was the head of Nurses on Wheels came to see me. He told me that I would get no more nursing support unless I stopped taking Nouss-Ade capsules. This visit occurred in about August 1998. By this time however I felt that I was totally cured. I had not been back to the hospital. I had no more heart problems so I felt that I did not need any more support from the Nursing service. I told him so but he did not seem to be interested."

"When I came to the last bottle of Nouss-Ade capsules that I had purchased in 1997 I wanted them to last so I reduced the dose

49

down to only 1 capsule per day. Then, when that bottle finally ran out I did not buy any more. Not long after I noticed that my energy level started to go down again, my heart problem returned and again I had problems in breathing. Dr. Owzinsky again put me back into Monash Hospital, this happened twice."

"So, in about December 1998 I again started to take Nouss-Ade capsules. That was when I found out that Nouss-Ade recommends that for people with pre-existing conditions, they should take 2 capsules in the morning and 2 capsules at night. This increase had an even greater affect on me:

The energy levels that I had years ago came back, I could work with no difficulty at all.

I had had difficulty in my ability to speak and this difficulty no longer exists, I am able to talk freely.

My ability to pay attention to detail has increased and I can now recall events, which before I had completely forgotten.

I am now driving again, with confidence and without difficulty, something that I have not done for years.

I have even noticed that the numbness in my feet is gradually going away.

50

I am now enjoying life and have commenced to study the Bible again."

"Most importantly, I use to have 1 injection of insulin ("26") in the morning and 1 injection of insulin ("16") in the evening but now, and for the last 5 months, I have not required any insulin injections at all. I monitor my blood sugar level and it has remained around 6~8. I no longer have any periods of sweating and I know my diabetes is totally under control."

Dysmenorrhea

Gay Sanders is a 43 year-old nurse. She says, "If I didn't take strong pain killers, I'd be rendered immobile with pain. I'd feel nauseated. My face would drain of all colour. This had been going on for years. At the first twinge of pain I'd begin to take Paradiene. I would continue to take 2 tablets every 4 hours for 2 days just to be able to function with daily life."

"For 3 months now I've been taking the Nouss-Ade capsules. Two months ago I decided to refrain from taking pain killer during menstruation. Aside from one single onset of pain, which woke me from sleep, I've had no pain at all. Perhaps twinges, but they remained twinges only."

"In comparison to the almost unbearable pain I had been suffering, this has been bliss. I have not taken strong pain killers for 2 months."

"In addition to this, my general stamina for the rigors of everyday living, recovery from stress + late nights has increased. Its as if life in that sense has smoothed out."

Prostate

Bob Yawie was diagnosed with prostate cancer for which his doctor prescribed a hormonal medication. "After three weeks of this medication I was feeling terrible, I had no feelings of any kind, was terribly short of breath + definitely should not have been driving (2 near accidents both my fault)."

After becoming aware of Nouss-Ade through a book on prostate cancer, Bob started on the product immediately. "After two months of your product I feel great, no longer short of breath even though I am still smoking (unfortunately). I now get up during the night for a piddle may-be once or twice. -Before: every hour."

"I don't know how the cancer is going but I have no pain in that area + seem to be regaining full sexual functions."

Another user, Geoff Muirden, reports, "Before taking Nouss-Ade I used to have to get up to relieve myself almost a dozen times a night, consequently I got little sleep. Thus ironically my problem was not inability to urinate, as explained in your book [Prostate: The Cure For Me], but excess ability to urinate."

"One week after taking Nouss-Ade I find I now need to get up at night only once or twice...."

Brian Oates writes, "I was diagnosed with Prostate Cancer in July 1997. My PSA count 221, in August I was operated on and they found that the cancer was in the right hand lymph nodes. As I could neither have Chemo or Radium treatment, I elected to have my testicles removed. They told me that I only had two years to live.

I started taking Nouss-Ade as soon as I came out of hospital and I have felt really well since, I put this down to the Nouss-Ade capsules. I have taken two capsules night and morning for the past year. After being on Nouss-Ade for the last twelve months, my PSA has now been lowered to 1. 9, and after another check-up, the Doctors have given Ten to Fifteen years."

Male Function

Raymond Wild of The Bowen Therapy Centre says Nouss-Ade is "Great for prostate and erection problems and general well being. No other product available as good."

Menopause

Jan Kena doesn't usually take supplements, but when her energy began to drop during menopause, she started trying lots of different products. "Nouss-Ade had the most natural effect for me, and I would recommend this product to anyone. My energy level was the first sign of change, making daily tasks achievable, and for all you women out there who have or are experiencing some form of menopause you would understand just what this means, an extra bonus was that I also lost weight through taking Nouss-Ade. I would personally recommend that when you buy Nouss-Ade for yourself, that you gift a bottle to someone dear to you, especially if they are looking for something natural, I can guarantee they will be back for more."

Uterus Cancer

Sharon was recovering from operations to remove her uterus and lymph nodes as well as from the effects of radiation therapy. Using naturopathic methods, she was still suffering both mentally and physically. She says, "1 week after being on Nouss-Ade...the remedy is everything you said it was.

I had a feeling of much more energy.

I needed less sleep.

I experienced a feeling of the "joy of life".

I was even "singing" around the house, something which has not happened for a long time.

I experienced a more "uncomplicated" outlook on life.

My metabolism changed and so did my diet. I particularly craved fruit and a lot of light cleansing foods.

The cold/flu life symptoms felt like they were beginning to break through after a couple of days and then they completely stopped.

My daily joint pains have gone away completely.

I did not develop neck & back problems during the week like I usually do.

My breathing capacity increased dramatically and found myself breathing clearly and deeply, without trying to do it.

My meditations improved dramatically, and felt I was able to 'tune in' again."

High Blood Pressure

Barry Grundler of Nauru has been on dialysis with blood pressures ranging between 160/110 and 140/100. He reports, "Well I am pleased to inform you that a week after taking Nouss-Ade (4 caps a day), I went to the hospital for my monthly check up and got an astonishing result for my blood pressure reading. In fact the sister was so shocked that she had to do three readings from the two machines and had received the same result, 120/80. After checking my medical file, last time I had such readings was 1993."

"Being an islander, I am a fisherman at heart and would normally fish nearly every day but due to arthritis my fishing days are limited and far between. Currently I'm on recreation leave and believe it or not, I'm now fishing almost daily. I'm still having

56

the occasional joint pains but are far less frequent than previously."

Psoriasis

Dr. Harry R. Alsleben reports, "My psoriasis lesions are still disappearing. Very impressive."

Skin Cancer

Wendy Lorger writes, "I am very pleased to tell you that our family has experienced various benefits from the capsules within one month. The most notable change has been with my brother. He had a very severe and painful skin cancer on his lip, which was very raw and was due to be cut out. After 3 weeks his lip cancer has all but dried up and disappeared. He also had a painful skin cancer on his ear and arm which have both dried up. He also has Hepatitis C, which we are very keen to have a blood test for in another 2 months to see if that has disappeared. He also had a cut at the corners of his mouth which he has had for 2 years, they have now disappeared."

"My brother is also a recovering alcoholic with a lot of liver damage, and we will also have that tested in 2 months. He has just started a full time job house painting and his boss is amazed at how much energy he has all day. He sleeps well for the first time in years. He is 48 years old."

"Myself, I am sleeping very well and eating a lot less. I am overweight and look forward to seeing the weight fall off after 3 months. I also had golden staph for 20 years and after one month has almost disappeared. I am so looking forward to the next few months."

"My son is 12 years old and was a healthy boy before Nouss-Ade, and his main improvement has been with a lot of mucous being expelled from his lungs. We are all going through a cleansing process and very regular at the toilet."

"My parents 80 years and 78 years old have been on it one month and have all the usual old age complaints, have not noticed any major change, except Mum had a rash on her body which has now disappeared."

Another happy customer, 49 year old Kimberly Rose, says, "I had many skin cancers on my hands and face which previously I have had burned off only to find that another crop pops up almost instantly. I have had a skin cancer on my left lower eye lid that could not be burnt off and so I was trying to find the courage to make the appointment to have it cut out and the others burnt off, once again."

"Imagine my surprise and joy when I realized that the cancer on my eye is gone and the many cancers on my hands and face are all but gone. Just one small cancer on each hand, and fading fast."

"I started taking Nouss-Ade almost twelve months ago now, because a friend thought it might help my immune system and give me more energy. At no stage did I hope that it would cure my skin cancers. I believed that the only way to manage them was to regularly have them burnt off and I was having the work done by people who are experts in the field."

"As well as taking Nouss-Ade, I have been taking some vitamin supplements, meditating and trying to clean up my act with regard to diet."

"This is very exciting but what is most exciting is the fact that if Nouss-Ade can make the skin cancers disappear just imagine what else it is repairing in the rest of my body."

Sleep

66 year-old Kathleen Ferguson writes, "the first things I was aware of after one week of taking Nouss-Ade was an innate feeling of well-being and lightness and I was having a very nurturing sleep...."

"Since taking Nouss-Ade I can honestly say that I am eliminating better and already losing weight gradually, actually breathing easier and deeper, tiredness minimal. I am much more alert, eating less, and feeling very well...."

"I think Nouss-Ade is wonderful, subtle yet very powerful in its healing."

"I have noticed that the surface veins on my legs are beginning to fade so I am truly happy with Nouss-Ade. Consequently I have been telling a few of my friends and acquaintances about it and a couple of them have started their own course of Nouss-Ade with so far excellent results."

Arthritis & Prostate Cancer

Anton Pallot is 57 years old. He writes, "About three years ago I was diagnosed with Arthritis and Prostate Cancer. The mental

60

stress that this caused was considerable. Physically I could not work, drive a car let alone walk. At times I could not go out and buy food. I had to sell my unit and financially I am still getting over these problems. Being told that I only had a few years to live caused me considerable stress and I needed counseling for months."

"Those who have arthritis will understand that the pain is nothing like any other. My hands, and knees in particular, would swell and at times it was impossible to pick up a mug of coffee. Fluid would be removed from one or both of my knees, 30cc plus each time. Now, as a consequence of taking Nouss-Ade capsules I am able to work as a security guard doing nightly 12-hour shifts. I still have a little pain when I arise in the morning; it disappears after I take the Nouss-Ade capsules. Yes, I get tired, but normally tired. I started work after I took Nouss-Ade capsules, I could not have worked prior to taking the capsules."

Anton continues, "The Nouss-Ade capsules are the only treatment I am having for the cancer, what I am doing is called Watchful Waiting against the specialist's recommendations. The problems I have had include considerable pain and difficulty in urinating. Frequently, if I need to pee, it was there and then, urgent and painful. My PSA, an antigen produced by the body that measures prostate cancer, went from normal "4" to 39.8" some 2 weeks ago it went down to 33.7. Most of the symptoms have now completely disappeared since I have started taking Nouss-Ade capsules."

"The day after I started on Nouss-Ade capsules I had a minor accident in the car. The people who were there with me, knowing my character, expected me to rant and rave. I didn't, since being on the capsules stress is there but I can handle it with ease…. Other areas I have noticed change is with my weight training, increased all weights, bulked up some and lost fat from the stomach. Skin damage from the sun on my arms has healed about 80%, so much so that my GP commented how good it looked. Sun tanning, I love it: I now tan without problems. I tried for three days not to take the capsules, all of the symptoms started coming back and I stressed out. So much so that those friends close to me, told me to get back on them!" Anton is now training to become a personal trainer, and plans to become a scuba instructor. "Prior to being on these capsules I physically could not have worked or contemplated doing these courses."

Tendonitis

Brenda suffered from chronic tendonitis of both forearms. Four cortisone injections had only worsened the condition, with acute attacks and daily spasms in both arms. After one week on Nouss-Ade, she reports, "I feel so wonderful it is just amazing. I cannot believe I feel so good in just one week. Everyone that sees me tells me I am looking so good, and asks me what I am doing!"

"My tendonitis has had no flare ups and the spasms have completely gone. My eyes feel clear and sparkling and I wake up in the morning feeling fresh and alive. I cannot believe how wonderful I feel."

"After a couple of days I gave up smoking cigarettes instantly and I also did not desire any alcohol. I had a small amount but it did not do anything for me. I felt better without it."

She reports, "After two weeks Nouss-Ade:

I have just had one of the best menstrual periods I have recalled in years.

Nous Energy

I had no headaches, no bloating, no stomach cramps, only slight breast tenderness as opposed to chronic engorged breasts usually. I also had no acne on my face and back.

All my previous cravings for sweets, sugary foods, confectionary, chocolates were gone.

I needed to eat less food because I did not feel as hungry. I was satisfied with natural foods and did not desire sweets, as a consequence I lost weight.

My eyes continued to become even more clear and sparkling and they felt like someone had washed them out with clear fresh water.

My breathing become very free and easy and I felt like a clear channel had been opened from my eyes down into my respiratory system."

Asthma

Oliver Stenning, age 13 writes, "Since taking 1 bottle (2 capsules morning and night after dinner) these are the changes that I have noticed.... I used to get Asthma when running around at my friends' houses, going to stuffy places and sleeping over at my friends. To help me with my asthma I needed my puffer. When I started taking Nouss-Ade capsules I notice that I hardly ever get asthma! I have not used my puffer since taking Nouss-Ade capsules, and I know that my asthma is going away."

"Hay fever is terrible! I get a blocked chest and a blocked nose. Whenever I slept over at people's places I got hay fever each time. Since I have been taking Nouss-Ade capsules I haven't got hay fever either. So I can now have sleep-overs...."

"I use to get constipation often, only going to the toilet once every 3 days, but since I have been taking Nouss-Ade capsules I go every day without constipation! I noticed this change within the first 3 to 4 days of starting the capsules."

"I always seem to have a runny nose, especially when I walk into the classroom, but now because of Nouss-Ade capsules I don't have a runny nose."

"I hate it when I get a head-ache or ear-ache, well, I haven't had either since taking Nouss-Ade capsules and I haven't had to take Panadol (drug), anymore also."

Ann Bennett writes, "My son Aaron is seven years old, and since he was six months old has been a chronic asthmatic. He has been taking steroid preventatives, ventolin and prednisolone (another steroid) to try to stay on top of his asthma. Aaron has also had to endure countless visits to hospital because of this horrible ailment. Since taking Nouss-Ade, I have gradually been dropping the dosage of his medication, and now he is not on anything at all. To date, Aaron has not had any symptoms or any signs of having an asthma attack which is of great relief to both himself and me. Also, towards the end of the year when most of his grade at school was off sick with the flu going around, Aaron was the only one that did not have time off for being sick. That in itself I found to be incredible as children pick up everything from each other.

As for myself, I started taking Nouss-Ade as I was always feeling tired. I would go to bed tired and wake up just as tired. My sleep patterns were terrible. I did not have trouble going to sleep, just staying asleep. As I was terribly run down, if there was a bug going around, I caught it. I felt like I was always at the doctors getting medicine for something or another. Now I sleep well, have more energy to cope with everything I do in a day, and reserves of energy to keep up the pace of a seven year old. I have found that I have not been sick at all and truly do feel that Nouss-Ade is a wonder product."

Migraine

Anthony Davies suffered migraine headaches since childhood, despite some help achieved through osteopathy, acupuncture and other treatments. Starting on 2 capsules a day of Nouss-Ade, he noticed some improvement, but continued getting occasional migraines. Since he has increased his dose to 3 capsules a day, he has not had one migraine in 6 months.

Herpes

Roy reports after 9 months on Nouss-Ade, "When I began taking the product I was not sick although I occasionally suffered from outbreaks of herpes. Within the first 2 weeks of taking the product I noticed that I had a few headaches, albeit mild ones, and I had quite a lot of flatulence."

"At the end of the first month I had a bad outbreak of herpes, although it went away completely in 3 days. Since then I have not had an outbreak. It would seem that it has gone away completely."

"During the second month I noticed that I was not hungry and I ate less. In fact, I began losing weight. The weight loss lasted for

3 months during which time I lost 9 kgs. I have kept the weight off. I made no attempt to diet, what I found was that I was not hungry very much. I ate 1 substantial meal a day, usually at night, during the day I ate 1 or 2 pieces of fruit, this was enough, I didn't get hungry."

"By the second month I noticed that my nails no longer developed the 'white spots' and my cuticles no longer tore or split. My hair seemed to grow very fast although this no longer occurs."

"The most noticeable change occurred in the third month, when I noticed my work-tiredness relationship changed. I noticed that I was not tired at all when I finished work at night. In fact now I work not less than 12 hours per day 6 days a week. My capacity to concentrate has also increased, over the 9 months this increase is dramatic although at the time, on a daily basis, the changes are subtle."

"During the 9 months I have had 1 mild cold, it lasted for 12 hours. I also got the flu. In the case of the flu, I noticed I had caught something when I awoke in the morning, slight sore throat, sneezing and headache. By 10 P.M. that night I was well and truly over it. The following day all that remained was a slight nasal congestion. I have not lost 1 day off work, working 6 days per week, in the last 9 months."

"The product is remarkable!"

Pain

A 61 year-old couple, Laurence and June Hoins have suffered from persistent and disabling bone and head pains, resorting to massive doses of aspirin for symptom relief. When the tried Nouss-Ade for 7 weeks, they report, "all of our painful symptoms disappeared, we didn't take one aspirin and we started to lose weight."

"We then stopped taking the capsules for a further six weeks and now, today, all of our painful symptoms have returned.... We will, therefore, now take these capsules every day of our remaining time on this planet."

Chronic Disease

Donna Lynch reports, "I have suffered with (8) chronic diseases most of my life.... Every kind of treatment available from anywhere in the world has been tried and failed. Partial success achieved only from HOMEOPATHY.... Now I am on my 4th bottle of Nouss-Ade and for the first time in my life can report steady improvement in all my conditions with" bipolar disorder and abuse patterns "now being completely cured!...Thank you very much for this product. I feel it working in my body, straightening, strengthening and freeing my mind. I've never been this clearheaded in my life. I look forward to whole health. Love, light + happiness (since taking Nouss-Ade)."

Nouss-Ade's ability to support the healing process from the energetic to the physical, from the spirit to the body is a marvelous indication of its true healing ability. In homeopathy, healing progresses from the mind to the body, and from deeper, more critical systems, to more superficial systems. By following these natural pathways, Nouss-Ade shows itself to be working with the body's own processes and priorities for restoration of total health. The body is designed to heal itself. It is designed to perpetuate life. It is divinely intelligent. Achieving maximum lifespan with optimum quality of health and life demands and deserves support with a product such as Nouss-Ade. Thank God its time has come.

Homeopathy & Retracing

In homeopathy, for over 200 years, physicians have observed the process of healing in minute detail. Retracing is a phenomenon in the natural history of healing where the body passes more or less briefly through symptoms similar to past disease states in the process of completing unfinished tissue detoxification and repair. Typically, this process also proceeds from more crucial, internal body areas outward, and downward from the head to the feet.

A Remission Foundation patron who started on Nouss-Ade as soon as it became available, Tina Stoeber, experienced this process first hand in a dynamic way. She reports, "The use of this product has been amazing. The first week using it therapeutically, my bowels began to work so well. Every time I ate I would eliminate. That was the first day. The second day I noticed a black glob in my fecal material that was flaky.

I was shocked, as the week progressed I kept having experiences of aches and pains around old injuries where I imagine there was scar tissue. Things seemed to move down, the ache or pain, until my feet hurt so bad I could barely walk. Then poof the next day it would completely disappear. When this happened in the beginning I became very tired and one weekend I slept almost 24 hours. Afterwards, I felt a sense of deep healing that was going on, healing my body systematically freeing me of old illnesses from my past one at a time, each one being brief and quickly exiting at my feet.

A heaviness I've felt in my head for a long time disappeared and I could breathe into my head. It was such a freeing experience that I felt I had an epiphany one night when I could not sleep at all. For three hours I was in what I call a bliss state where I knew that my body was healing itself so that I could do the work I came here to do. I was having an experience of being able to take in energy from the air, the rain, the trees. Could this product also be awakening a spiritual part of my being? It could very well have been a contributing factor.

I don't drink alcohol or take any drugs or smoke anything and haven't for almost 18 years. I am a vegetarian also for the same # of years and have had difficulty since menopause with extra abdominal weight and a great appetite sometimes for things better not eaten like sweets. My cravings seem to be disappearing and I don't need to eat so much. I eat better and eat less food.

I did not change anything else in my vitamins or lifestyle or exercise. I already exercise five days a week, doing yoga and aquaerobics. That is one reason I think it is working so fast,

72

because I move my body. Yet dare I say cure-all. I am amazed and can't wait to see what happens next, since my energy is now going up & up. My mind is clearer and I am so happy. I want to share this product with everyone I know."

Longevity

Kevin Sweeney writes, "I have been taking it for a little over two months now and the results are amazing! I feel younger, stronger, and much more able to cope with the stresses of everyday living and I can feel my body changing in every way for the better....

After a few weeks on the product I was able to pass three kidney stones that had been bothering me for years. The CAT Scan is clear with no more stones in sight. The amazing thing was how good I felt the next day. The first time I passed stones, before taking Nouss-Ade I was laid up for several days afterwards. This time I was at the gym the second day feeling great! Just recently a skin cancer that I would have normally had burned off, just fell off my arm. I also cannot find a large mole that used to be on my scalp.

I am sleeping less, waking feeling more refreshed, eating less and loving life more and more. Joint pain is almost non-existent. I do get a minor headache now and then but I can feel that is due to the detoxifying going on. My skin is better, my eyes are clearer and I feel an absence of any kind of physical problem. It feels like every organ is operating the way it should. At the gym now the muscle seems to be coming back faster than ever with less effort.

I'm planning to stay on this one forever and get younger as time goes on."

Outro

Long after the original publication of this book, a very significant research study has been completed recently by retired University of Calgary Professor Carmen Boulter. She measured the body's energy field and the chakras before, during and after exposure to the nouss energy field inside the great pyramid of Giza.

Before entering the pyramid, the body's energy field was not significantly connected with any of the chakras. There was correlation between Chakras 5 & 6 at a significance level of $p < 0.001$, between Chakras 2 & 6 at $p < 0.05$, and between Chakras 1 & 2 at $p < 0.01$. I would read this as the visitors being grounded and oriented to their spatial and social milieu.

Inside the pyramid, the only significant inter-Chakra correlation was between Chakras 6 & 7 at $p < 0.05$. This, I would read as a transcendental spiritual focus on the divine and cosmic realms. The body's energy field meantime was fired up!

Chakra 1: $p < 0.05$

Chakra 2: $p < 0.01$

Chakra 3: $p < 0.001$

Nous Energy

Chakra 5: $p < 0.05$

Chakra 7: $p < 0.001$

Thus, all but Chakras 4 & 6 are showing coherent activity inside the pyramid. I read the most significant activity ($p < 0.001$) as an expression of the Divine Will (Chakras 7 & 3). This correlates the visions shown to Luisa Piccarreta (1865-1947), known as the Little Daughter of the Divine Will, for the energetics of this new cycle of Time.

The observed after-effects are equally enlightening. Chakra connections abound:

Chakras 1 & 6 at $p < 0.01$

Chakras 2 & 7 at $p < 0.01$

Chakras 3 & 4 at $p < 0.05$

Chakras 4 & 6 at $p < 0.05$

Thus, all but Chakra 5 show functional inter-linkage in this mode of being, which I read as being a state of integrating the nouss energy effects, which appears to be a speechless state beyond words, beyond description at least in that time frame. The personal sphere of spiritual activity centered on the Heart, Chakra 4 links down to Chakra 3 (will) and up to Chakra 6 (vision), which then links down to Chakra 1 (grounding). Chakra 2 (social) & 7 (divine) show as a second circuit of transpersonal spiritual activity.

At the same time, the body's energy field is showing coherence in the heart and vision centers:

Chakra 4: $p < 0.001$
Chakra 6: $p < 0.01$

Note that these are precisely the only areas that did not show such activity while inside the pyramid! The most significant activity is centered in the Heart, the fire in the middle! And in Oriental Medicine that is where the Shen, the Spirit, resides. And it is seen in the eyes! Always interesting...

Afterward

Now that Nouss-Ade has opened a sort of reverse Pandora's Box of healing and related questions, there is no putting it back in that black box of the unconscious. Spiritual healing and knowledge always seem to open more doors and conceptual spaces to explore than they fully illuminate. I hope this little collection of observations and thoughts will fuel further useful contemplation and exploration by you dear reader...

Conclusion

Nouss-Ade has been and continues to be, so long as precious supplies last, a real problem solver in the healing process of the whole being, mind, body and spirit. In God's economy, such Graces show up precisely how they are needed, or rather, precisely how they are able to be received, utilized and appreciated.

I remain grateful that such an energy as that found qualitatively, and identified quantitatively by the inventor, Andrew Savva, at the Giza Pyramids, has found its way home to 19.47 degrees North Latitude, the Earth's Heart Center in Hawai'i... by way of a resonance point in the Australian desert...

The angels are busy... even as we sleep.

Postscript

A dozen years after putting this little monograph together, I find myself reprinting it here, because time has proven it to continue being worthy of continued attention. Precious samples of Nouss-Ade stored near 19.47 degrees latitude in Hawai'i have shown zero aging or deterioration of any kind. They appear to contain an immortal energetic quality. Their clinical and spiritual healing efficacy is undiminished, undiluted by the river of time. This kind of temporal coherence is a sign of the life of the spirit, just as the bodies of certain Saints are found to be incorrupt, as was the case with our own blessed Father Damien of Molokai, and prior to that, of Kalapana. When his body was removed from these beloved islands where his spirit intended it to remain, it lost its incorruptible quality, as if some remaining coherence of his spirit in that former biological vessel had deigned to leave at that time.

Glossary

AGE: Advanced Glycation Endproducts are the damaging result of excess sugars binding to the body's tissues.

Anti-oxidant: by definition this is an electron donor. The most efficient source of electrons is to ensure we are connected to them from the earth, and are supplying them in abundance in the air and water. This preserves nutritional anti-oxidants for their important co-enzyme functions.

Avascular: lacking a direct blood supply. The interior tissues of the eye, and even the macula lutea in the central retina, in order to be optically clear lack blood vessels once the tissue develops in utero. The remnants of the hyaline artery, active during gestation, cast shadows on the retina, called muscae voluntantes (physiological floaters).

Brunescent: a yellowing of the crystalline lens of the eye.

BEV: see Bio-electronics of Vincent

Bio-Electronics of Vincent (BEV): BEV is an objective means of measuring and calculating energy based on both the electrical (electron) and magnetic (proton) factors in addition to the energetic information factor (photon) via ion content or conductivity (the inverse of resistivity). BEV measurement and analysis can be applied to blood, urine, saliva, water, nutrients, or other substances via measurement of the standard physical parameters: pH, rH2 or O.R.P., and resistivity.

Biokinesiology: Biokinesiology is an advanced method of muscle testing which integrates biocommunication protocols from European electro-dermal testing (see Vegetative Reflex Test and Electroacupuncture According to Voll).

Cataract: a loss of clarity of the crystalline lens of the eye. Clarity of the lens is one of the best known predictors of longevity.

Carrier frequency: A carrier frequency is the frequency or rate at which an oscillating pattern repeats. It acts as the carrier of the information contained in the characteristic pattern of the waveform. The carrier determines the energy content of the individual photons, which transmit the wave. Each specific carrier frequency is like a different AM (amplitude modulation) radio station.

Characteristic waveform: The characteristic waveform is the shape of an electromagnetic oscillation. It is determined by its specific source and represents information content of the electromagnetic oscillation. A characteristic waveform is like the programming on a radio station.

Ciliary Body: the nearest circulation to the lens of the eye, and thus its remote source of nutrition. Like the joints, the lens itself is an avascular tissue.

Crystalline Lens: the lens in the eye that is the densest protein in the body, the most exposed tissue to ionizing radiation, and particularly sensitive to oxidation by free radicals and glycation by sugars (producing AGE), two of the dominant processes of unhealthy aging.

Dowsing: Dowsing is an ancient art of finding water or other substances through amplification of subtle body responses. Dowsers may use wooden or metal dowsing rods, a pendulum, radionic instruments or other convenient amplification devices.

Dry Eye Syndrome: Most often a lack of mucin, the protein which makes the cornea wettable. This is stimulated by Vitamin A, which can be supplied directly in the form of eye drops. More severe cases often involve metal toxicity as well.

Dysbiosis: an imbalance in the normal flora of the body. The body is not a sterile monoculture, but a symbiotic polyculture, right down to the mitochondria, an intracellular bacterium inherited exclusively through the maternal line.

Electroacupuncture According to Voll: EAV is a form of electrodermal remedy testing developed in 1953 by Rheinhold Voll, a German dentist and medical doctor. This system allows the measurement of points and meridians that correspond to specific internal body organs and functions.

Electromagnetic: Electromagnetic field radiation is composed of electrical, magnetic and information components. Electrostatic fields are produced by stationary electrical charges, such as the capacitor in a television set (even when unplugged). Magnetic fields are produced by electrical charges in constant motion, as in a direct current. When electrical charges change their pattern of motion, as in alternating current, electromagnetic radiation is produced. Information is carried in carrier and characteristics waveforms as well as scalar (information only) waves.

Electronic factor: The concentration of electrons in a fluid medium, such as in all biological systems is one of 3 factors, which determine biological energy via the Nernst equation. The other two factors are the magnetic factor and the ion content (electrical conductivity). Because free electrons quickly combine with free protons to produce hydrogen (H_2), their concentration is measured as a function of hydrogen molecules (rH_2).

Fovea Centralis: normally the point of maximum visual clarity, except in night vision, since there are no rod cells in the macular area.

Glaucoma: Wrongly defined as high pressure in the eyes (IOP) even by most physicians, since a high percentage of glaucomatous eyes actually have low pressure. Glaucoma has many patterns related to nutritional deficiencies and toxicities, but is ultimately the result of damage to the optic nerve.

Healing Crisis: this can be a flu-like reaction observed when taking a stimulatory medicine such as homeopathy. It can be based in a cleansing or detoxification reaction, eliminating stored toxins, or can be a Herxheimer, or die-off process, eliminating bacterial endotoxins or other wastes in the case of dysbiosis.

Hertz: The number of oscillations per second of an electromagnetic field is given the unit Hertz (Hz).

Homeopathy: Homeopathic substances are produced by successive dilution and succussion, resulting in increasing potencies containing increasing electromagnetic carrier frequencies and decreasing chemical concentrations.

Homotoxicology: Homotoxicology is the study of toxins in man. As toxins penetrate further into the system, they may enter more vital organs and tissues. They may also interfere at deeper levels within the cell and ultimately the nucleus. The reversal of this process is marked by a shift in symptoms to more superficial or less vital areas according to anatomy and histology. This detoxification process may also be marked by local metabolism of toxins accompanied inflammatory symptoms, and by increased elimination through mucus membranes, skin, urine or feces.

Homeopathy: the leading form of medicine in the world today in terms of numbers of people treated, and a non-toxic medicine, free of side effects, that works by hormesis, stimulating the body to heal itself by recruiting pathways of response that have been dormant, often due to adaptation to past stresses. Modern science is finally catching up with the field of epigenetics. For over 200 years doctors in this field have watched the non-genetic inheritance of miasms.

Hormesis: The law of dosage effect in pharmacology, also known as the Arndt-Schultz law. Small doses stimulate the body's healing mechanisms. Moderate doses irritate and suppress the ability of those pathways to produce a functional response. Larger doses destroy the same cells.

Ion: A positively or negatively charged particle is an ion. Ions are capable of carrying electrical energy within the body by their movement. The total ion concentration determines the electrical conductivity of a fluid, which is one of 3 factors determining the total energy content according to the Nernst equation. The other two are the electrical and the magnetic factors.

IOP: Intra-Ocular Pressure. High pressure is always an issue, but low or normal pressure does not guarantee health eye tissues and good visual function.

Macula Lutea: the yellow spot in the center of the retina is avascular tissue at the center of which is the Fovea Centralis,

91

normally the point of maximum visual clarity, except in night vision, since their are no rod cells in the macula. The macula has the highest oxygen demand of any tissue in the body, and is energetically linked to the lungs.

Magnetic factor: The concentration of protons, which are positively charged ions, is measured by the magnetic factor (pH). It is one of the 3 basic factors, which determine the amount of biological energy via the Nernst equation. The other factors are the electrical factor and the ion content or electrical conductivity.

Mitochondria: supply 90% of the healthy cell's energy through aerobic metabolism via the electron transport chain, which relies on the B Vitamins as co-factors, and on Oxygen to receive the spent electrons once energy has been extracted for storage and use as ATP.

Muscae Voluntantes: The remnants of the hyaline artery, active during gestation, cast shadows on the retina, as physiological floaters. Toxins in the colon and food reactions can make this shadow darker and more annoying.

Multi-dimensional: Multi-dimensional refers to any process, which has more than just one or two dimensions or key factors.

In truth, everything is multi-dimensional. It is only our limited perception, representation or thinking about something that can appear linear (1D) or flat (2D). Space is multi-dimensional (3D). Space-time, which Einstein conceived to be inseparable except by the perception of each individual observer, is 4D. Physicists may now view the universe as 6D, I0D or 26D depending on the context and model proposed.

Pendulum: A pendulum is a simple device consisting of a suspended weight used to amplify subtle neuromuscular patterns in the arm for the detection of biological responses to subtle electromagnetic energy fields.

PSC: Posterior Subcapsular Cataract. This is often a fast onset cataract affecting younger people than most other types. It often relates to immune function and typically responds very well to certain remedies including TMG and Cernilton Flower Pollen.

Radiesthesia: Radionics is an approach to detection of biological responses to subtle electromagnetic energy fields using a stick-plate, which is rubbed by the fingertips. Amplification of subtle physiological changes takes place via noticeable changes in the feel and sound of the stickiness of the stick-plate. Numbers called rates may be used to identify various fields, just as these fields might be identified by names or by numbers such as frequencies, wavelengths, or other characteristics of an electromagnetic oscillation.

Retracing: the tendency to reverse the steps of disease, only much faster in most cases, in the course of the healing process.

Soil Based Organisms (SBO): providing enzyme systems for detoxification, biological transmutation of elements and other functions to assist in altering the course of chronic health issues.

Spectroscopy: A spectroscope measures the intensity of different frequencies of electromagnetic radiation. It is not able to measure the characteristic waveforms of the radiation. The information provided by spectroscopy is therefore like knowing what channels are on the air, but not being able to identify the programming. The most sensitive indicators of the characteristic information in electromagnetic radiation are the physiological responses of biological systems.

Strabismus: an eye that turns in a different direction than its fellow eye. Typically eyes turn in with an increase in acidity that causes increased muscle tension in the extra-ocular muscles, since the Medial Rectus muscles have the largest cross sectional diameter. When the metabolism becomes blocked by an even larger accumulation of the toxin, the pH swings to alkaline, and muscle tone drops below normal, resulting in an outward eye turn. In the course of restoring healthy function, it is often observed that the outward tendency (exo) will convert to inward (eso) on its way to restoring balance. This reversal of the pathway of disease in the healing process is called the eso-exo swing in this context, and in general is a form of retracing.

Vegatetative Reflex Test: Formerly called the Vegatest Method, developed in 1979 by Dr. Helmut Schimmel, this is a method of electronic monitoring of skin resistance at an acupuncture point. Homeopathic stimuli are used to determine the patterns of causality and relief from stress at that time.

Vincent: see Bio-electronics of Vincent

Vitreous Body: the jelly like substance filling the back part of the eye, behind the lens. This is where most floaters occur. The vitreous is energetically linked to the large intestine.

Bibliography

Alternative Medicine: The Definitive Guide (Compiled by The Burton Goldberg Group, Future Medicine Publishing, Inc., Puyallup, Washington, 1993).

Balch JF and Balch PA. Prescription for Nutritional Healing. Garden City Park, NY: Avery Publishing Group, 1990.

Berridge EW. Diseases of the Eyes. Jain Publishers, New Delhi, 1984.

Brinker F. Herb Contraindications and Drug Interactions (Eclectic Medical Publications, Sandy, Oregon, 1998).

Burr HS. Blueprint for Immortality: The Electric Patterns of Life (C. W. Daniel Co. Ltd., Saffron Walden, England, 1972).

Chidre D, and Martin H with Beech D. The Heartmath Solution (HarperSanFrancisco, 1999).

Deville M. The Real Trace Element Problem: Their Therapeutic Applications (Centre de Recherches et d'Applications sur les Oligo-Elements).

Nous Energy

Dinshah D.   Let There Be Light (Dinshah Health Society, Malaga, New Jersey, 1985).

Duke J.   Dr. Duke's Phytochemical and Ethnobotanical Databases are online at http://ars-grin.gov/duke/

Gerber R.   Vibrational Medicine: New Choices for Healing Ourselves (Bear & Company, Santa Fe, New Mexico, 1988).

Grossman, M and Swartwout G.   Natural Eye Care, An Encyclopedia: Complementary Treatments for Improving and Saving Your Eyes (Keats Publishing, Los Angeles, 1999).

Hahnemann, S. Organon of Medicine (J. P. Tarcher, Inc. , Los Angeles, 1982, translated from original written by Samuel Hahnemann 1755—1843.

Hollwich, F.   The Influence of Ocular Light Perception on Metabolism in Man and in Animal (Springer Verlag, New York, Heidelberg, Berlin, 1979).

Jackson M and Teague T.   The Handbook of Alternatives to Chemical Medicine.   (Oakland, California: Teague and Jackson, 1985)

Kappel G. Nutrition and Vision, OEP Foundation, Santa Ana, Calif. 1980.

Kavner RS and Dusky L. Total Vision, (AW Visual Library, New York, 1978).

Kenyon, JN. Modern Techniques of Acupuncture: A Scientific Guide to Bioelectronic Regulatory Techniques and Complex Homeopathy (Thorsons Publishing Group, Wellingborough, England, 1985).

Kervran CL. Biological Transmutations (Beekman Publishers, Inc. , New York, 1971; originally published in French by L Courrier du Livre, 1966).

Kutsky RJ. Handbook of Vitamins, Minerals and Hormones (Van Nostrand Reinhold Company, New York, 1981).

Lane B. Nutrition and Vision, 273-274, in Bland J, Ed. 1984-85 Yearbook of Nutritional Medicine (New Canaan, Connecticut: Keats, 1985).

Mandel P. Energy Emission Analysis: New Applications of Kirlian Photography for Holistic Health (Synthesis, W Germany)

Mandel P. Practical Compendium of Colorpuncture (Energetik Verlag, Bruchsal, W Germany, 1986).

Manning CA and Vanrenen LJ. Bioenergetic Medicines East and West: Acupuncture and Homeopathy (North Atlantic Books, Berkeley, California 1988).

Moffat JL. Homoeopathic Therapeutics in Ophthalmology. Jain Publishers, New Delhi, 1982.

Murphy R. Homeopathic Medical Repertory: A Modern Alphabetic Repertory (Hahnemann Academy of North America, 1993).

Norton AB. Ophthalmic Diseases and Therapeutics. Jain Publishers, New Delhi, 1987.

Ober C, Sinatra ST, and Zucker M. Earthing: The most important health discovery ever? (Basic Health Publications, Inc., Laguna Beach, California, 2010).

Oschman JL. Energy Medicine: The Scientific Basis (Churchill Livingstone, an imprint of Harcourt Publishers Ltd, 2000).

Page LR. Healthy Healing. (Sacramento, California: Spilman Printing, 1990)

Pearson D and Shaw S. Life Extension, A practical scientific approach, (Warner Books, New York, 1983).

Pischinger A. Matrix and Matrix Regulation: Basis for a Holistic Theory in Medicine (Haug International, Brussels, 1991, 1st German edition 1975).

Pizzorno JE and Murray MT. A Textbook of Natural Medicine. Seattle, WA: John Bastyr College Publications, 1987.

Randolph TG and Moss RW. An Alternative Approach to Allergies (Bantam Books, New York, 1980).

Sardi B. Nutrition and the Eyes. (Montclair, California: Health Spectrum Publishers, 1994)

Shils ME, Olson JA and Shike M. Modern Nutrition in Health and Disease, Eighth Edition (Williams & Wilkins, Media, PA, 1994).

Smith CW and Best S. Electromagnetic Man (St. Martin's Press, New York, 1989).

Spitler HR. The Syntonic Principle: Its Relation to Health and Ocular Problems (College of Syntonic Optometry, Eaton, Ohia, 1941).

Nous Energy

Stortebecker P. Dental Caries as a Cause of Nervous Disorders (Stortebecker Foundation for Research, Stockholm, Sweden, 1982).

Stortebecker P. Mercury Poisoning from Dental Amalgam - A Hazard to Human Brain (Stortebecker Foundation for Research, Stockholm, Sweden, 1985).

Swartwout GM. Biofields: The New Physics of Health.

Swartwout GM. Electromagnetic Pollution Solutions: What You Can Do To Keep Your Home and Workplace Safe.

Swartwout GM. Glaucoma Solutions: Prevention and Reversal.

Swartwout GM. Vision for Living, 1983.

Todd GP. Nutrition, Health & Disease. Norfolk, Virginia: Donning Co. , 1985.

Valnet J. The Practice of Aromatherapy: A Classic Compendium of Plant Medicines &Their Healing Properties (Healing Arts Press, Rochester, Vermont, 1980, English translation 1982).

Voll R. 2nd Supplement to the Four Volume Work: Topographical Positions of the Measurement Points of Electroacupuncture According to Voll. EAV Diagnosis of Eye
102

Diseases, 15 New Measurement Points for Portions of the Eye, EAV Therapy for Eye Diseases, 5 New Approaches. Medizinisch Literarische Verlagesellschaft MBH, Uelzen, 1983.

Werbach MR, Murray MT. Botanical Influences on Illness. Tarzana, California: Third Line Press, 1994.

Whang S. Reverse Aging: Scientific Health Methods Easier and More Effective than Diet and Exercise (Siloam Enterprises, Englewood Cliffs, NJ, 1994).

Wurtman RJ, Baum MJ, and Potts JT. The Medical and Biological Effects of Light (The New York Academy of Sciences, New York, 1985).

About the Author

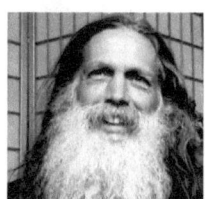

Rev. Dr. Glen Swartwout graduated Magna Cum Laude with honors in Environmental Earth Sciences and Chemistry from Dartmouth College, and received his doctorate at the top of his class in Vision Science with honors in Optics as well as Leadership, being inducted into both Beta Sigma Kappa and the Gold Key Honor Societies at the State University of New York in Manhattan, where he trained at the largest outpatient vision clinic in the world. He served as Editor, Vice President and President of the American Optometric Student Association serving 4000 international student doctor members. He is the author of over 50 professional papers, books, and software programs. His first professional office was in Tokyo, Japan.

Nous Energy

Also by this author

Cataract Solutions: Prevention & Reversal Via Accelerated Self-Healing

Electromagnetic Pollution Solutions

Biofields: The New Physics of Health

Healing Glaucoma

Macular Degeneration... ...Macular Regeneration

The Shire: Cultivating Your Future Self

Materia Medica: Vis Medicatrix Naturae

Refreshing Vision: Opening the Windows of the Soul

More writings by this author

http://christiascelli.wordpress.com

http://doctorglen.wordpress.com

http://pahoasark.wordpress.com

http://selfgrowth.com/articles/user/240198

Additional contributions by this author

Alternative Medicine, The Definitive Guide (contributor)

EPFX SCIO QXCI Quantum Xeroid Eclosion Consciousness Interface (contributor)

IBIS: Interactive BodyMind Information System (contributor)

Natural Eye Care, An Encyclopedia (co-author with Marc Grossman, O.D., L.Ac.)

Connect online

Website: http://drglen.weebly.com

About.me: http://about.me/drglen

Facebook: http://facebook.com/DrSwartwout

LinkedIn:
http://www.linkedin.com/pub/glen-swartwout/10/902/5aa

Twitter: http://twitter.com/DoctorGlen

YouTube: http://youtube.com/doctorglen

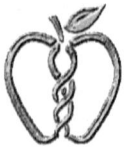